Cop)

Contents

What It Is..6

How does the Ornish Diet Work? 7

What You Can Eat..11

The Ornish Lifestyle Medicine Dietary Guidelines
....16

Eat Mostly Plants in Their Natural Form 17

Limit Empty Carbs: 18

Four Grams a Day of Healthy Fats..............19

Eat Mostly Plant-Based Proteins.................20

Limit Sodium...22

Reduce Caffeine Intake..............................22

Pros and Cons 24

Pros 24

Cons 27

The Ornish Diet Sample Menu Plan 30

Spectrum prevention plan 30

Spectrum reversing-heart-disease plan 32

ORNISH DIET RECIPES 34

Ornish Apple Spice 34

Ornish Cocoa Truffles 37

Ornish Chocolate Pudding 41

Ornish White Bean and Winter Green Soup 43

Ornish White Bean and Carrot Soup 46

Ornish Moroccan Vegetable Stew Recipe 49

Ornish Reversal Hummus Recipe 53

Healthy Pizza Pasta Salad 55

Black Bean and Corn Salad 58

Ornish Breakfast Quinoa Recipe 60

Ornish Apple Spice Muffins 63

Ornish Eggplant Parmesan............................67

Ornish Traditional Split Pea Soup..................73

Ornish Spinach, Apple and Fennel Salad.........76

DEAN ORNISH'S GRANOLA 79

Ornish Caesar Salad 81

Ornish Fast and Sloppy Joes 84

Ornish Pasta Carbonara..............................88

Banana Rice Pudding 92

1-2-3 Tasty Morning Scramble 94

Ornish Egg White and Vegetable Frittata 95

Ornish Tofu Teryaki 100

Lentil Soup 104

Ornish Carrot Cupcakes with Non-fat Maple frosting 107

Ornish Mac 'n Cheez 111

Un-Do It Tacos............................... 115

Ornish Lentil Loaf 118

Pumpkin Pie................................. 122

Ornish Edamole............................. 127

Ornish Spinach and Mushroom Egg White

Scramble Recipe........................... 129

What It Is

The Ornish Diet was created in 1977 by Dr. Dean Ornish to help people "feel better, live longer, lose weight and gain health," and consists of three major components: nutrition, stress management, and exercise.

In terms of nutrition, the diet recommends low-fat, plant-based foods, such as:

- Fruits

- Vegetables

- Whole grains

- Legumes

- Soy products

- Nonfat dairy products

- Egg whites in their natural form (not packaged liquid egg whites)

- Good fats that contain omega-3 fatty acids

Unlike many other diet fads, the Ornish Diet does not solely focus on what you eat, rather emphasizing the importance of exercise, stress management, and relationships in addition to the foods on your plate.

How does the Ornish Diet Work?

Along with changes in nutrition, the Ornish diet involves making changes to your lifestyle, such as prioritizing exercise, improving stress management, and fostering strong and healthy relationships, in order to make a beneficial impact on your health and well-being.

Ornish categorizes food into five groups, also known as a "spectrum," from healthiest (Group 1) to least healthy (Group 5). Each group within the spectrum consists of different guidelines:

- Group 1: Predominately fruits and vegetables, whole grains, legumes, and nonfat dairy products.

- Group 2: Consists of mainly plant-based foods, however there is an increase in monosaturated and polyunsaturated fats, otherwise known as "healthy" fats. These foods include avocados, seeds, nuts, and canola oil.

- Group 3: Includes some seafood, such as salmon, and reduced-fat dairy products.

- Group 4: Consists of foods that have fewer nutrients and more fat, as well as anima products. Poultry, whole milk and dairy products, mayonnaise, pastries, and cookies are all examples of foods within Group 4.

• Group 5: The end of the spectrum and least healthy, Group 5, is highest in saturated fat and trans fatty acids, or unhealthy fats. This group consists of fried foods, red meat, along with many other high-fat foods.

Based on your health needs and goals, you can find where you are on the spectrum and make changes to your diet as you see fit.

When it comes to fitness, Ornish emphasizes regular, moderate exercise, prioritizing aerobic activities, resistance training, and flexibility. Ornish encourages a minimum of 30 minutes a day or an hour every other day of aerobic activities, along with resistance or strength training 2-3 times per week. Whether you are following a diet plan or not, regular exercise, in big or small increments, can lead to substantial long-term benefits, such as preventing chronic diseases and promoting mental health and well-being.

Stress management can be a difficult task for many, however finding self-care practices that work for you and setting aside time each day can make a significant impact on your mental and physical health. There are many ways to manage stress, such as deep breathing, meditation, or yoga. If you find yourself needing additional help, Health Coaches are available to work with you in order to effectively manage stress and prevent it from standing in the way of your goals.

What You Can Eat

Ornish counsels that we will find success not by restricting calories, but by watching the ones we eat. He breaks this down into foods that should be eaten all of the time, some of the time, and none of the time.

The following can be eaten whenever you are hungry, until you are full:

• Beans and legumes

• Fruits -- anything from apples to watermelon, from raspberries to pineapples

• Grains

• Vegetables

These should be eaten in moderation:

- Nonfat dairy products -- skim milk, nonfat yogurt, nonfat cheeses, nonfat sour cream, and egg whites

- Nonfat or very low-fat commercially available products --from Life Choice frozen dinners to Haagen-Dazs frozen yogurt bars and Entenmann's fat-free desserts (but if sugar is among the first few ingredients listed, put it back on the shelf)

These should be avoided:

- Meat of all kinds -- red and white, fish and fowl (if we can't give up meat, we should at least eat as little as possible)

- Oils and oil-containing products, such as margarine and most salad dressings

- Avocados

- Olives

- Nuts and seeds

- Dairy products (other than the nonfat ones above)

- Sugar and simple sugar derivatives -- honey, molasses, corn syrup, and high-fructose syrup

- Alcohol

- Anything commercially prepared that has more than two grams of fat per serving

That's it. If you stick to this plan, you will meet Ornish's recommendation of less than 10% of your calories from fat, without the need to count fat grams or calories. Ornish suggests eating a lot of little meals because this diet makes you feel hungry more often. You will feel full faster, and you'll eat more food without increasing the number of calories.

Ornish's regimen is more than mere diet, he claims. He is a stickler about incorporating at least 30 minutes of moderate exercise a day, or an hour three times a week, and using some kind of stress-management technique, which might include meditation, massage, psychotherapy, or yoga.

Fruits and Vegetables

This diet is vegetarian, so prepare for plenty of produce. In addition to those fruits and veggies, you will use vegetarian sources of fats, such as olive oil, for cooking.

Whole Grains

On this diet, you must swap refined carbohydrates for whole grain versions—so, whole-wheat bread instead of white, for example.

Legumes, Seeds, and Nuts

Legumes are a good source of protein in a plant-based diet. More nuts and seeds are available on the prevention plan.

Meat, Poultry, and Fish

On the reversal Ornish diet, no animal proteins are allowed, since they contain saturated fats. On the prevention plan, some fish is included since it is a good source of omega-3 fatty acids.

Eggs

Egg whites are permitted, but not yolks, because of their cholesterol content.

Dairy Products

Small amounts of nonfat milk or yogurt are allowed.

The Ornish Lifestyle Medicine Dietary Guidelines

Where some diets focus on food restrictions, the Ornish Diet does not focus on counting calories or tracking your nutrient intake. Although there are suggestions for nutrition that are encouraged, the diet can be done in moderation.

In general, the Ornish Diet is low-fat, plant-based diet, and predominately consists of fruits, vegetables, whole grains, legumes, soy products, nonfat dairy, and egg whites, as well as healthy fats such as foods with omega-3 fatty acids. According to Ornish, the diet emphasizes real foods as they're found in nature rather than processed foods, along with fiber and many complex carbohydrates.

Ornish dietary guidelines is as follows;

Eat Mostly Plants in Their Natural Form

Plant-based foods include:

- Fruits

- Vegetables

- Whole grains

- Legumes

- Non-fat dairy foods (no more than two servings/day)

- Egg whites

Ornish recommends small, frequent meals spread throughout the day in order to maintain or reach a healthy body weight and keep energy levels constant.

Limit Empty Carbs:

The Ornish Diet does not ban sugar intake; however, it is not encouraged. The guidelines recommend limiting added sugars, non-fat sweets, and refined carbohydrates to no more than two servings/day. Bad carbs include foods such as:

- Refined white flour and white rice

- Concentrated sweeteners

- Processed foods such as chips

Alcohol is also not encouraged but is allowed in limited amounts. If alcohol is consumed, only one serving per day (1.5 ounces of liquor, 4 ounces of wine or 12 ounces of beer) is recommended.

Four Grams a Day of Healthy Fats

An important aspect of the Ornish Diet is that it is very low-fat, with a nutrition plan having no more than ten percent of calories being from fat. These calories from fat should come from fats found in whole foods.

According to the Ornish Diet, healthy fats include:

• Fish oil

• Flax seed oil

- Plankton-based omega-3 fatty acids

- Small amounts of nuts and seeds

Ornish also notes limiting cholesterol to 10 milligrams or less per day. Instead of using non-fat dairy products, you can also use nondairy products, which tend to be cholesterol-free.

Due to the high concentration of fat in nuts, they are only allowed in small amounts, with the suggestion of three or less servings per day. However, specific nuts and seeds contain antioxidants and cardio-protective phytochemicals that contribute to cardiovascular health benefits. For example, studies have shown that almonds lower LDL cholesterol and protect heart health.

Eat Mostly Plant-Based Proteins

Eating plant-based proteins instead of animal products will not only avoid consuming high amounts of saturated fats and cholesterol, but also lower your risk of heart disease, diabetes, and obesity. Even though animal products, such as poultry, are not restricted, Ornish encourages followers to stick to plant-based proteins.

Plant-based proteins include:

- Egg whites

- Tofu

- Tempeh

- Beans

- Legumes

- Non-fat yogurt

- Non-fat cheese

Limit Sodium

The Ornish Diet recommends using spices, herbs, and other natural flavors, such as citrus and vinegars, to flavor food instead of salt. According to the American Heart Association, eating less sodium can significantly lower your risk for high blood pressure, which is the highest risk factor for heart disease, as well as reduce bloating.

Reduce Caffeine Intake

Reducing the intake of stimulants such as caffeine can lead to a more balanced, calm and peaceful way of living, according to Ornish. For this reason, the Ornish Diet discourages drinking coffee and limiting intake to one cup or less of coffee, up to two cups of decaf, or up two cups of black tea per day.

Although caffeine can lessen fatigue, speed up metabolism and often improve your mood, there are also adverse effects. Caffeine increases your heart rate and causes a quick spike in blood pressure, which are risks the Ornish Diet aims to avoid completely by partaking in this diet.

Starting a new diet and making changes to your nutrition may seem overwhelming at first, however the Ornish Diet encourages each follower to make choices based on personal preference and at a pace comfortable for them.

If you are looking to start the Ornish diet, check out these healthy recipes, like a Lotus Stem

Salad, Dairy-Free Berry Vanilla Soft-Serve, or a Vegan Chickpea Omelet.

Pros and Cons

Like many other diet plans, the Ornish Diet has benefits, as well as downsides.

Pros

The Ornish Diet may be associated with several health benefits.

May aid weight loss

The Ornish Diet emphasizes nutrient-dense ingredients like fruits, veggies, and plant-based proteins, making it an excellent option if you're looking to lose weight.

According to one study in 20 people, following the Ornish Diet for 1 year resulted in an average weight loss of 7.5 pounds (3.3 kg), which was greater than other popular diets like Atkins, Weight Watchers, and the Zone Diet.

Similarly, another 1-year study found that 76 participants who followed the Ornish Diet lost an average of 5 pounds (2.2 kg).

Furthermore, other studies show that switching to a vegetarian diet could aid weight loss.

In one study in 74 people with type 2 diabetes, following a vegetarian diet for 6 months was significantly more effective than a low-calorie diet at promoting fat loss.

Aids disease prevention

Promising research suggests that the Ornish Diet could help prevent chronic disease.

In fact, studies show that vegetarian diets may be associated with a lower risk of heart disease, diabetes, and obesity.

Other studies have found that vegetarian and vegan diets may be linked to a lower risk of certain types of cancer, including stomach, colorectal, prostate, and breast cancer.

What's more, one small study in 18 people compared the effects of three popular diets, including the Ornish Diet, over 4 weeks.

The Ornish Diet reduced levels of total cholesterol, triglycerides, LDL (bad) cholesterol, and inflammation, all of which are risk factors for heart disease.

Flexible and easy to follow

Unlike other diet plans that require you to carefully count calories or track your nutrient intake, the Ornish Diet requires minimal effort and is relatively easy to follow.

According to the diet's creator, aside from certain animal products, no foods are completely off-limits on the plan — though some ingredients should be limited.

Even certain prepackaged convenience items like veggie burgers or whole-grain cereals are permitted in moderation, provided they contain fewer than 3 grams of fat per serving.

Given that the diet is not overloaded with complicated rules and regulations, it's easy to stick to in the long run.

Cons

Though the Ornish Diet is associated with several potential benefits, there are some downsides to consider.

For starters, it's very low in healthy fats, with less than 10% of total daily calories coming from fat.

Most health experts and regulatory agencies recommend getting around 20–35% of your total daily calories from fat to help optimize health.

Healthy fats like mono- and polyunsaturated fatty acids can protect against heart disease, reduce inflammation, support brain function, and ensure healthy growth and development.

Additionally, it's important to keep in mind that removing meat and certain animal products from your diet can increase your risk of nutritional deficiencies.

In fact, studies show that vegetarian diets tend to be lower in important nutrients like protein, calcium, vitamin B12, and zinc.

Monitoring your intake of these key vitamins and minerals and enjoying a variety of nutrient-dense fruits, veggies, whole grains, and legumes can ensure that you're able to meet your needs while following the Ornish Diet.

You may also opt to take a multivitamin, which can help fill any gaps in your diet to prevent a nutritional deficiency.

The Ornish Diet Sample Menu Plan

Here are two days of typical meals, both between 1,800 and 1,900 calories. The first menu is based on foods from Ornish's three healthiest food groups (out of five he divides foods into); the second is his plan to reverse heart disease. You can find recipes for these meals on the Ornish website.

Spectrum prevention plan

Breakfast

2 egg-white vegetable scramble.

1/3 cup each blueberries, strawberries and raspberries.

1/2 cup nonfat milk.

1 slice whole-grain bread.

Lunch

1 1/4 cup roasted-tomato soup

2 1/2 cups Asian noodle salad topped with 5 grilled shrimp

1 slice whole-wheat peach griddle cake

Snack

2/3 ounces dark chocolate

3 apricots

10 raw almonds

1/2 cup plain nonfat yogurt

Dinner

3-ounce wild salmon

1 1/4 cup butter lettuce/pear salad with honey-infused vinaigrette

1 1/2 cup sweet corn, black bean and tomato salad

5/8 cup peach bread pudding

Glass of wine or sparkling water

Spectrum reversing-heart-disease plan

Breakfast

1 3/4 egg-white zucchini frittata

1/3 cup each blueberries, strawberries and blackberries

1/2 cup nonfat milk

1 slice whole-grain bread

1 cup tea or decaf coffee

Lunch

1 7/8 cup mango-beet salad

1 7/8 cup vegetarian chili

1 slice corn bread

Snack

5/8 cup green pea guacamole

6 whole-wheat pita bread wedges

1/2 cup red grapes

Dinner

1 7/8 cup fennel and arugula salad with fig vinaigrette

2 cups whole-wheat penne pasta with roasted vegetables

2 1/3 cup fruit-and-yogurt trifle

Glass of wine or sparkling water

ORNISH DIET RECIPES

The following recipes are psoriasis diet-friendly while also being a treat to the taste buds. Try some of these psoriasis diet recipes today.

Ornish Apple Spice

Preparation time

45 minutes

INGREDIENTS

1. Nonstick cooking spray

2. 2 CUPS whole wheat flour or gluten-free flour blend

3. ½ CUP old-fashioned rolled oats

4. ½ CUP flax meal

5. 2 TEASPOONS pumpkin pie spice (see Chef's Note)

6. 1 TEASPOON baking powder

7. 1 TEASPOON baking soda

8. ½ TEASPOON fine sea salt

9. ½ TEASPOON stevia powder

10. 1 ¼ CUPS unsweetened applesauce

11. ½ CUP apricot fruit spread (fruit juice-sweetened only)

12. 1 CUP apple grated about 1 medium apple

13. 1 CUP chopped dried apple

14. ½ CUP raisins

15. 2 TEASPOONS vanilla extract

Instructions

- Preheat oven to 350ºF.

- Spray a 12-cup non-stick muffin pan lightly with cooking spray, or line muffin pan with paper liners and spray liners lightly with cooking spray.

- In a medium bowl, whisk together whole wheat flour or gluten-free flour blend, oatmeal, flax meal, pumpkin pie spice, baking powder, baking soda, salt, and stevia powder.

- In a large bowl, stir together the applesauce, apricot fruit spread, grated apple, dried apple, raisins, and vanilla extract.

- Stir in half the dry ingredients, then stir in the remaining half until just mixed.

- The mixture may look lumpy.

- Spoon one-third cup batter into each muffin cup.

- Bake the muffins until a toothpick comes out clean from the center of a muffin, about 35 minutes. Be careful not to overcook.

- Place muffin pan on a rack and let cool for 10 minutes, until muffins pull away slightly from the edges of the muffin cups.

- Remove muffins from pan. Serve warm or let cool on a rack to room temperature.

Ornish Cocoa Truffles

Preparation time

15 minutes

INGREDIENTS

- 1 CUP FRESH pitted medjool dates firmly packed about 9 dates, or 6 oz

- ½ CUP unsweetened cocoa powder (suggested brand: Hershey or Green & Black 100% cacao powder)

- 1 ½ TEASPOONS vanilla extract

- ¼ TEASPOON fine sea salt

- ½ TEASPOON cinnamon (optional: for Mexican Truffles)

- 1/8 TEASPOON cayenne pepper (optional: for Mexican Truffle)

- ¼ CUP unsweetened cocoa powder (optional: for rolling)

- ¼ CUP turbinado (raw) sugar (optional: for rolling)

Instructions

1. Place dates in a small bowl.

2. Cover with hot water and let soak for 15 minutes. Drain and pat dry.

3. Using a food processor fitted with a metal blade, pulse dates several times to make a paste. Add cocoa powder, vanilla, and salt.

4. To make Mexican Truffles, add cinnamon and cayenne. Pulse 3 or 4 times (mixture will seem dry).

5. Add 1 tablespoon warm water, and pulse several more times, adding another tablespoon of warm water if mixture still seems dry.

6. Continue to pulse until mixture is smooth and forms a ball.

7. Remove truffle mixture from processor and transfer to a bowl.

8. Put ¼ cup cocoa powder or turbinado (raw) sugar in a shallow bowl. Using 1 tablespoon of truffle mixture for each ball, shape balls between the palms of your hands. (If mixture seems sticky, refrigerate until well chilled before rolling.) Roll each ball in cocoa powder or sugar after shaping.

9. Cover and refrigerate until serving.

Ornish Chocolate Pudding

Preparation time

5 minutes

INGREDIENTS

- 16 OZ firm silken tofu patted dry 2 cups

- ¾ CUP unsweetened cocoa powder (suggested brand: Hershey's)

- ¼ CUP pure maple syrup

- ¼ CUP water

- 1 TABLESPOON pure vanilla extract

- 1 ½ TEASPOONS powdered stevia

- PINCH fine sea salt

- 1 CUP raspberries or chopped strawberries garnish, optional

Instructions

1. In the bowl of a food processor fitted with a metal blade, combine tofu, cocoa powder, maple syrup, water, vanilla extract, stevia, and salt. Process until mixture is smooth and creamy, stopping as necessary to scrape down sides and center of the bowl with a rubber spatula.

2. Taste and adjust seasoning as needed with more maple syrup and/or vanilla.

3. Adjust consistency with a little more water as needed.

4. Divide pudding mixture between 6 small serving dishes. Refrigerate until chilled, about least 30 minutes.

5. Top each portion with berries, if using.

Ornish White Bean and Winter Green Soup

Preparation time

40 minutes

INGREDIENTS

- 1 ½ CUPS onion coarsely chopped

- 2 TEASPOONS garlic minced

- 4 CUPS low-sodium vegetable broth, divided

- 3 CUPS cooked cannellini or navy beans or two 15-oz cans cannellini or navy beans, rinsed and drained

- 2 CUPS sweet potatoes peeled and coarsely chopped

- 3 TABLESPOONS sweet white miso

- 2 TEASPOONS fresh thyme, divided chopped

- ¼ TEASPOON fine sea salt

- ¼ TEASPOON freshly ground pepper

- 2 CUPS FIRMLY PACKED kale or chard tough ribs removed, roughly chopped

- 1 ½ oz Crushed red pepper flakes (optional)

Instructions

- In a 3-quart saucepan over medium heat, combine onion, garlic, and ½ cup of the broth.

- Cook, stirring frequently, until onions are softened and transparent, about 10 minutes.

- Add the remaining 3 1/2 cups of broth, beans, sweet potatoes, miso, 1 1/2 teaspoons of the thyme, salt and pepper.

- Bring to a simmer and cook until sweet potatoes are tender and flavors have melded, about 10 to 15 minutes.

- Add kale and remaining ½ teaspoon thyme.

- Simmer until kale is tender, about 3 to 4 minutes.

- Taste for seasoning, adding more miso or pepper as needed.

- Sprinkle with crushed red pepper flakes before serving, if desired. This soup is best made one to two days in advance; cover and refrigerate until needed.

Ornish White Bean and Carrot Soup

Preparation time

1 hour 15 minutes

INGREDIENTS

1. 2 CUPS dry white beans such as Great Northern, cannellini, or navy

2. 7 CUPS low-sodium vegetable broth

3. 1 bay leaf

4. 3 CUPS carrots peeled and diced

5. 2 CUPS onions peeled and diced

6. 1 TABLESPOON garlic pressed or minced

7. 1 TABLESPOON fresh thyme chopped or 1 teaspoon dried

8. 1 TABLESPOON fresh marjoram or oregano chopped or 1 teaspoon dried

9. ¼ TEASPOON fine sea salt

10. ¼ TEASPOON freshly ground pepper

Instructions

- In a medium bowl, cover beans with cold water by several inches. Let soak for at least 8 hours or overnight.

- Drain the soaked beans, discarding soaking liquid. In a large pot over high heat, combine beans with vegetable broth and bring to a boil.

- Skim off any foam that forms on the surface.

- Reduce heat to medium-low.

- Add bay leaf. Partially cover and let simmer, stirring occasionally, for 15 minutes.

- Add carrots, onions, garlic, thyme, marjoram, salt, and pepper. Let simmer, partially covered, until beans are tender, about 45 minutes Remove from heat.

- Remove bay leaf and discard.

- Measure out 2 cups of the cooked beans along with ½ cup of the cooking liquid.

- Place beans and cooking liquid in a blender. Blend until smooth, adding additional cooking liquid if necessary.

- Return bean puree to the remaining beans and liquid in the pot and stir to combine.

- Taste for seasoning, adding additional salt and/or pepper as needed. Reheat as necessary for serving.

Ornish Moroccan Vegetable Stew Recipe

Preparation time

1 hour 20 minutes

INGREDIENTS

1. 2 CUPS onion peeled and diced

2. 2 TEASPOONS garlic pressed or minced

3. 1 ½ TABLESPOONS fresh ginger root peeled and finely chopped

4. 2 TEASPOONS ground coriander, divided

5. 1 cinnamon stick, about 3" long

6. ½ TEASPOON turmeric

7. ¼ TEASPOON fine sea salt

8. 3 ½ CUPS low-sodium vegetable broth

9. 3 CUPS butternut squash peeled and chopped (1 lb)

10. ONE 14.5-OZ CAN fire-roasted diced tomatoes (suggested brand: Muir Glen)

11. 2 CUPS green beans cut to 1-in lengths (½ lb)

12. 1 ½ CUPS cooked garbanzo beans (chickpeas) or one 15-oz can, rinsed and drained

13. ½ CUP golden raisins firmly packed

14. ZEST OF 1 lemon

15. ½ CUP cilantro chopped

16. 1 ½ CUPS cooked quinoa warmed (FOR SERVING)

Instructions

1. In a large, 4 quart saucepan over medium heat, combine onions, garlic, ginger, 1 1/2 teaspoons of the coriander, cinnamon stick, turmeric, and salt with 1/2 cup of the vegetable broth.

2. Sauté, stirring frequently, for 7-10 minutes, until onions are softened and translucent.

3. Add remaining 3 cups vegetable broth, butternut squash, and tomatoes. Increase heat to high and bring to a boil.

4. Reduce heat to medium and simmer for about 30 minutes, until squash is just barely cooked through.

5. Add green beans, garbanzo beans, raisins, and lemon zest. Cook for 7-10 minutes, until green beans are tender.

6. Stir in remaining ½ teaspoon coriander.

7. Just before serving, stir in cilantro.

8. Serve warm, over quinoa.

Ornish Reversal Hummus Recipe

Preparation time

5 minutes

INGREDIENTS

1. 3 CUPS cooked garbanzo beans (chickpeas) or two 15-oz cans no salt added garbanzo beans, rinsed and drained

2. ½ CUP water

3. 1 ½ TABLESPOONS lemon juice

4. 2 TEASPOONS ground cumin

5. 1 ½ TEASPOONS ground coriander

6. 1 TEASPOON garlic finely chopped or pressed

7. ½ TEASPOON fine sea salt

8. ¼ TEASPOON freshly ground pepper

9. 1/3 CUP cilantro leaves, firmly packed finely chopped

10. 2 TABLESPOONS mint leaves chopped

11. Paprika for garnish

Instructions

- Place garbanzo beans, water, lemon juice, cumin, coriander, garlic, salt, and pepper in a food processor fitted with a metal blade.

- Process until smooth and creamy, adding more water as needed to achieve desired consistency.

- Add cilantro and mint.

- Pulse briefly to incorporate; herbs should "speckle" the mixture rather than turn it completely green.

- Spoon hummus into a serving bowl. Sprinkle with paprika before serving.

Healthy Pizza Pasta Salad

Preparation time

30 minutes

INGREDIENTS

1. 16 oz gluten-free pasta (2 8-oz boxes)

2. 1 15-oz can chickpeas or cannellini beans, rinsed and drained

3. 1 15-oz can kidney beans, rinsed and drained

4. 1 large green bell pepper (or 2 small), seeded and diced

5. 1 c julienned sun-dried tomatoes, lightly packed (see note)

6. ½ c pitted black olives, sliced

7. ⅔ c fat-free or lite Italian dressing (DIY version here)

8. 2 tsp dried oregano leaves

9. ¼ c toasted pine nuts (omit to keep McDougall-friendly)

Instructions

• Cook pasta according to directions on package.

• While pasta is cooking, toss remaining ingredients in a large bowl, reserving 1 Tbsp of pine nuts.

• When pasta is cooked, rinse with cold water and immediately add to salad. Toss gently to coat.

• Top with remaining 1 Tbsp pine nuts.

Black Bean and Corn Salad

Preparation time

15 minutes

Ingredients

1. 2 cans of black beans, drained and rinsed well (or 3 cups cooked)

2. 1 can fire roasted, diced tomatoes 15 oz

3. 1 package of frozen corn, 16 oz., thawed by running under warm water in drainer

4. 1/2 purple onion, diced

5. 1 can of water chestnuts, drained and rinsed 8 oz

6. bunch cilantro, chopped (1/4 cup or more)

7. 2 Tbsp lime juice

8. zest from 1 lime

9. 3 + Tbsps. balsamic vinegar, to suite your taste

10. Salt and garlic powder, to your taste

Instructions

1. If using canned black beans, drain and rinse them before using them. To do this, I pour them into a colander and rinse under warm water.

2. Next, place the frozen corn in the colander and run the kernels under warm water to defrost. There is no need to cook it.

3. Dice the purple onion and chop up the cilantro.

4. For the lime, I recommend using a citrus zester to zest it before squeezing out the juice for this recipe. When it's whole, it is much more firm and easy to zest.

5. Combine all ingredients in a large bowl and mix well. The recipe calls for 3 tablespoons of balsamic vinegar, but I love balsamic and actually use a little more.

6. Stir together thoroughly and serve.

7. This tastes even better after a few hours (or next day) after marinating in the refrigerator.

Ornish Breakfast Quinoa Recipe

Preparation time

20 minutes

INGREDIENTS

For Quinoa:

1. 1 CUP white quinoa

2. 2 CUPS water

3. 1/3 CUP golden or dark raisins

4. PINCH fine sea salt

For Porridge:

- 1 ½ CUPS unsweetened soy milk

- 2 TEASPOONS vanilla extract

- ½ TEASPOON powdered stevia (optional)

- ½ TEASPOON pumpkin pie spice or cinnamon (see Chef's Note)

- PINCH fine sea salt

Instructions

1. 1. Using a fine-mesh strainer, rinse quinoa well.

2. 2. In a small 1½ quart heavy-bottomed saucepan, combine quinoa, water, raisins, and pinch of salt.

3. Over high heat, bring to a boil.

4. 3. Reduce heat to a simmer, cover, and cook until all water is absorbed, about 10 to 15 minutes.

5. 4. While quinoa is cooking, whisk together the soy milk, vanilla, stevia if using, pumpkin pie spice or cinnamon, and a pinch of salt in a medium bowl.

6. 5. Stir soy milk mixture into the quinoa.

7. Let simmer, stirring occasionally, until mixture is heated through, 1–2 minutes.

8. Divide into 6 bowls.

9. Sprinkle with additional pumpkin pie spice or cinnamon.

10. Serve warm.

Ornish Apple Spice Muffins

Preparation time

45 minutes

INGREDIENTS

Nonstick cooking spray

1. 2 CUPS whole wheat flour or gluten-free flour blend

2. ½ CUP old-fashioned rolled oats

3. ½ CUP flax meal

4. 2 TEASPOONS pumpkin pie spice (see Chef's Note)

5. 1 TEASPOON baking powder

6. 1 TEASPOON baking soda

7. ½ TEASPOON fine sea salt

8. ½ TEASPOON stevia powder

9. 1 ¼ CUPS unsweetened applesauce

10. ½ CUP apricot fruit spread (fruit juice-sweetened only)

11. 1 CUP apple grated about 1 medium apple

12. 1 CUP chopped dried apple

13. ½ CUP raisins

14. 2 TEASPOONS vanilla extract

Instructions

• Preheat oven to 350ºF.

• Spray a 12-cup non-stick muffin pan lightly with cooking spray, or line muffin pan with paper liners and spray liners lightly with cooking spray.

- In a medium bowl, whisk together whole wheat flour or gluten-free flour blend, oatmeal, flax meal, pumpkin pie spice, baking powder, baking soda, salt, and stevia powder.

- In a large bowl, stir together the applesauce, apricot fruit spread, grated apple, dried apple, raisins, and vanilla extract.

- Stir in half the dry ingredients, then stir in the remaining half until just mixed. The mixture may look lumpy.

- Spoon one-third cup batter into each muffin cup.

- Bake the muffins until a toothpick comes out clean from the center of a muffin, about 35 minutes. Be careful not to overcook.

- Place muffin pan on a rack and let cool for 10 minutes, until muffins pull away slightly from the edges of the muffin cups.

- Remove muffins from pan. Serve warm or let cool on a rack to room temperature.

Ornish Eggplant Parmesan

Preparation time

2 hours

INGREDIENTS

For Eggplant:

- ½ CUP egg whites from 4 eggs

- ¼ TEASPOON fine sea salt

- 1 ¼ CUPS fat-free, whole-grain (or gluten-free) breadcrumbs

- 2 small to medium eggplants cut into 1/2-in slices (about 16 to 20 slices total) see Chef's Note

For Filling:

1. 1 LB frozen spinach thawed

2. 8 OZ firm tofu patted dry and finely crumbled

3. ¾ TEASPOON garlic powder

4. ¾ TEASPOON onion powder

5. ¼ TEASPOON fine sea salt

6. 1/8 TEASPOON freshly ground pepper

For Assembly:

- ONE 24-OZ jar low-fat marinara sauce

- 1 CUP fat-free mozzarella cheese shredded (optional)

- ¼ CUP fresh basil chopped

Instructions

1. Preheat oven to 375ºF. Line a baking sheet with parchment paper.

2. Place egg whites and ¼ teaspoon salt in a small, shallow bowl.

3. Whisk vigorously with a fork until light and frothy.

4. Place breadcrumbs in a second small shallow bowl.

5. One slice at a time, dip eggplant into the egg whites, coating each side.

6. Then, dip each slice into the breadcrumbs, coating each side.

7. Press the crumbs onto each slice as necessary to make them stick. (So your hands don't get gloppy, use one hand to dip the eggplant into the egg whites and the other to dip into the crumbs.)

8. Place crumb-coated eggplant slices on the prepared baking sheet.

9. Bake until eggplant slices are cooked through and lightly brown on top, about 35 minutes.

10. Remove the eggplant from the oven.

11. While eggplant is baking, make the filling.

12. Place thawed spinach in a colander in the sink or over a deep bowl.

13. Using your hands, squeeze or press spinach vigorously to remove excess liquid.

14. Continue to squeeze and press spinach until it is almost dry.

15. After draining, you should have about 1½ cups of spinach.

16. In a medium bowl, stir together the drained spinach, finely crumbled tofu, onion powder, garlic powder, 1/4 teaspoon salt and pepper. Set aside.

17. To assemble the eggplant parmesan, spread 1 cup of marinara sauce evenly over the bottom of a 9 x 13-in glass Pyrex baking dish. Arrange 8 to 10 of the baked eggplant slices on top of the marinara.

18. Spoon 1/3 cup of the spinach mixture on top of each piece of eggplant. Top each piece of eggplant with a heaping tablespoon of marinara sauce.

19. Top each eggplant slice with another, similarly-sized slice of eggplant, lightly pressing the slices together.

20. Spoon the remaining marinara sauce over the eggplant slices. Sprinkle slices with cheese, if using. (Recipe can be prepared up to this point, 1 to 2 days in advance. Cover and

refrigerate until needed. Preheat oven to 375ºF before baking.)

21. Bake the eggplant parmesan until eggplant and filling have heated through and cheese has melted, 30–35 minutes.

22. To brown top, increase oven heat to broil. Move baking dish to the upper third of the oven, about 6 to 8 inches below the heat. Broil for one to two minutes, until the top is lightly browned and bubbly. Remove from the oven. Sprinkle with basil just before serving.

Ornish Traditional Split Pea Soup

Preparation time

1 hour

INGREDIENTS

1. 2 CUPS split peas, green or yellow rinsed (12 oz)

2. 8 CUPS water

3. 2 CUPS red-skinned potatoes coarsely chopped (12 oz)

4. 2 CUPS onion peeled and coarsely chopped

5. 1 ½ CUPS carrots peeled and coarsely chopped

6. 1 ½ CUPS celery coarsely chopped

7. 2 TABLESPOONS garlic pressed or minced

8. 1 TABLESPOON fresh oregano or 1 teaspoon dried

9. 1 TABLESPOON fresh rosemary or 1 teaspoon dried

10. 1 TABLESPOON fresh thyme or 1 teaspoon dried

11. 1 ½ TEASPOONS Better than Bouillon No-Beef Base

12. 1 TABLESPOON sherry vinegar

13. ½ TEASPOON natural liquid smoke (optional)

14. ½ TEASPOON fine sea salt

15. ½ TEASPOON freshly ground pepper

Instructions

• In a large, heavy-bottomed pot over high heat, combine all ingredients and bring to a boil.

- Reduce heat to medium and simmer, stirring occasionally, until peas are very soft and vegetables are tender, 35–45 minutes.

- Taste for seasoning, adding additional vinegar, salt and/or pepper as needed.

Ornish Spinach, Apple and Fennel Salad

Preparation time

15 minutes

INGREDIENTS

For Vinaigrette:

1. 4 TABLESPOONS apple cider vinegar preferably raw, unfiltered, organic

2. ½ TEASPOON orange zest

3. 1 TABLESPOON fresh orange juice

4. 1 ½ TEASPOONS pure maple syrup

5. 1 TEASPOON whole grain mustard

6. ½ TEASPOON ground fennel seeds

7. ½ TEASPOON curry powder

8. ¼ TEASPOON freshly ground pepper

9. ¼ TEASPOON fine sea salt

For Salad:

8 CUPS baby spinach

- 2 apples cored and thinly sliced such as Braeburn, Honeycrisp, or Pink Lady

- 1 medium sized fresh fennel bulb, about 8 oz cored and thinly sliced (2 cups)

- 1/3 CUP dry roasted soy nuts (see Chef's Note)

- ¼ CUP scallions chopped

Instructions

1. To make the vinaigrette, in a small bowl, whisk together apple cider vinegar, orange zest, orange juice, maple syrup, grainy mustard, ground fennel, curry powder, salt, and pepper. Set aside.

2. In a large bowl, toss the spinach with the apples, fennel, soy nuts, and scallions.

3. Season lightly with additional salt and pepper, if desired.

4. Toss with three-quarters of the vinaigrette.

5. Taste for seasoning. Add remaining vinaigrette as necessary. Serve immediately.

DEAN ORNISH'S GRANOLA

Preparation time

2 hours

INGREDIENTS

- 2 cups rolled oats

- 1/4 cup oat bran

- 1/2 cup rye flakes

- 2 tablespoons soy crumbles, See NOTE

- 1/4 cup apple juice

- 1 teaspoon vanilla

- 1 teaspoon ground cinnamon

- 1/2 teaspoon fresh grated nutmeg

- 1/4 cup dates, chopped and pitted

- 1/4 cup raisins

Instructions

- Mix everything but the dates and raisins and toss to cover with the apple juice.

- Bake for 1 1/2 to 2 hours at 300°F

- Cool; add dates and raisins.

- Place in airtight containers in a cool place

Ornish Caesar Salad

Preparation time

35 minutes

INGREDIENTS

For Dressing:

- 6 OZ silken tofu drained

- 2 TABLESPOONS water

- 2 TABLESPOONS fresh lemon juice

- 1 TABLESPOON red wine vinegar

- 1 TABLESPOON capers rinsed and drained (optional)

- 1 ½ TEASPOONS vegan Worcestershire sauce

- 1 ½ TEASPOONS prepared horseradish

- 1 TEASPOON garlic pressed or minced

- 2 TABLESPOONS nutritional yeast

- 1 TEASPOON dry mustard powder such as Coleman's

- ½ TEASPOON onion powder

- ¼ TEASPOON salt

- 1/8 TEASPOON freshly ground pepper

For Salad:

1. 4 SLICES whole grain bread or 1 ½ cups packaged fat-free croutons

2. 8 CUPS romaine lettuce torn or roughly chopped

3. 2 carrots peeled and thinly sliced

4. ½ CUP radishes thinly sliced

Instructions

1. To make the dressing, in a blender, combine tofu, water, lemon juice, red wine vinegar, capers, if using, Worcestershire sauce, horseradish, garlic, nutritional yeast, mustard powder, onion powder, salt, and pepper.

2. Blend on high speed for about 10 seconds, until mixture is smooth. (Dressing can be

prepared several days in advance and refrigerated until needed.)

3. If making croutons, preheat oven to 250ºF. Line a baking sheet with parchment paper. Trim crusts from bread slices. Cut bread into 1-inch cubes (or preferred crouton size). Spread on prepared baking sheet. Bake until crisp throughout, about 15 to 20 minutes. Let cool.

4. In a large bowl, combine romaine lettuce, carrots, radishes and croutons, if using. Add half of the dressing. Toss and taste for seasoning. Add additional dressing as needed. Serve immediately.

Ornish Fast and Sloppy Joes

Preparation time

5 minutes

INGREDIENTS

1. ONE 12-OZ PACKAGE vegetarian ground-meat alternative (suggested brand: Yves Veggie Ground or Lightlife Smart Ground)

2. 1½ CUPS cooked pinto beans or one 15-oz can, rinsed and drained

3. ½ CUP prepared barbecue sauce

4. 1/3 CUP tomato paste

5. 2/3 CUP water

6. ¼ CUP green onions (scallions) chopped

7. 2 TEASPOONS apple cider vinegar

8. ½ TEASPOON smoked paprika

9. ¼ TEASPOON freshly ground black pepper

10. 6 whole-grain buns (less than 3 grams of fat, with 3 grams or more of fiber)

11. ¾ CUP nonfat cheese, such as Monterey Jack or mozzarella shredded (optional)

12. ¼ CUP green onions (scallions) chopped for garnish

Instructions

- In a medium saucepan over medium heat, combine ground meat alternative, pinto beans, and barbecue sauce. In a small bowl, whisk together tomato paste and water until smooth. Add tomato paste to bean mixture along with ¼ cup green onions, apple cider vinegar, smoked paprika, and pepper.

• Reduce heat to low and cook, stirring occasionally, until mixture is warm and flavors have melded, 5-7 minutes. While filling is cooking, toast buns.

• To serve as a closed sandwich, spoon ½ cup filling onto bottom half of bun. Top with 2 tablespoons grated nonfat cheese and a sprinkle of green onions, if using. Top with top half of bun. To serve open faced, spoon ¼ cup filling over each half of bun. Top each half with 1 tablespoon nonfat grated cheese and a sprinkle of green onion, if using.

Ornish Pasta Carbonara

Preparation time

30 minutes

Ingredients

1. 6 OUNCES uncooked whole grain or gluten-free penne pasta (2 cups)

2. 2/3 CUP frozen baby peas

3. 2 CUPS broccoli florets (5 oz)

4. ¼ CUP dried tomatoes not oil-packed

5. 2 CUPS unsweetened low-fat soy milk

6. ¼ CUP Roasted Garlic puree (see description, above, for link)

7. 2 TABLESPOONS white miso

8. 1 ½ TABLESPOONS nutritional yeast

9. 1 ½ TEASPOONS fresh oregano finely chopped or ½ teaspoon dried

10. 1 TEASPOON chipotle pepper in adobo sauce

11. 1 TEASPOON sweet paprika

12. 2 TEASPOONS arrowroot, cornstarch, or sweet rice flour

13. 1 TABLESPOON water

14. Fine sea salt to taste

- Freshly ground pepper to taste

Instructions

- Fill a large saucepan two-thirds full of water.

- Bring to boil over high heat.

- Cook pasta according to package directions. One minute before pasta is ready, add peas.

- Drain pasta and peas in a colander and set aside.

- While pasta is cooking, place a vegetable steamer basket in a saucepan and add water to just below bottom of steamer basket. Over medium heat, bring water to a boil. Add broccoli.

- Cover and steam until broccoli is just tender but still bright green, 4 to 5 minutes.

- Remove basket from steamer and set aside.

- In a small bowl, cover dried tomatoes with hot water.

- Let stand until tomatoes are softened, about 5 minutes. Drain. Slice tomatoes into strips.

- In a medium-sized, heavy-bottomed saucepan over medium heat, whisk together soy milk, roasted garlic, miso, nutritional yeast, oregano, chipotle pepper, and paprika. Add drained tomato and bring mixture to a simmer.

- Cook, whisking frequently, until mixture starts to thicken, 4–5 minutes.

- In a small bowl, whisk arrowroot with 1 tablespoon water to make a smooth paste. Whisk paste into sauce and cook until mixture thickens, 1–2 minutes.

- Just before serving, stir pasta, peas, and broccoli into sauce. Cook, stirring, until mixture is heated through. Taste for seasoning, adding salt and/or pepper as needed. Serve immediately.

Banana Rice Pudding

Preparation time

1 hour

INGREDIENTS

- 1 1/2 c Brown rice; cooked

- 1 md Banana; cut in slices

- 1/2 ts Ground nutmeg

- 1 cn Fruit; (15-ounce can), cut in slices

- 1/4 c Water

- 1 ts Pure vanilla extract

- 1 c Nonfat milk

- 2 tb Honey

- 1/2 ts Ground cinnamon

INSTRUCTIONS

1. In a medium-size saucepan, combine the banana and fruit slices, water, honey, vanilla, cinnamon and nutmeg.

2. Bring to a boil, reduce the heat, and simmer for 10 minutes, or until quite tender but not mushy.

3. Add the rice and milk and mix thoroughly .

4. Bring to a boil and simmer 10 more minutes.

5. Serve warm.

1-2-3 Tasty Morning Scramble

Preparation time

10 minutes

Ingredients

1. 2 large egg whites beaten

2. 1 pinch granulated garlic

3. 1 bunch baby spinach

4. 1/4 c chopped tomato

5. 1 pinch fresh pepper

Instructions

- Spray a non-stick pan with non-stick cooking spray.

- Add spinach.

- After spinach begins to wilt add eggs, garlic and salt and pepper.

- Continue stirring the eggs until cooked.

- Top with tomato.

Ornish Egg White and Vegetable Frittata

Preparation time

40 minutes

INGREDIENTS

- 2 CUPS white mushrooms thinly sliced

- 4 oz

- 1 CUP zucchini coarsely chopped

- 1 CUP yellow onion diced

- ½ CUP dried tomatoes cut into thin strips

- 1 TABLESPOON fresh thyme, divided chopped

- 2 TEASPOONS garlic pressed or minced

- ½ TEASPOON fine sea salt

- ½ TEASPOON freshly ground pepper, divided

- ½ CUP water

- 2 CUPS kale finely chopped

- 2 CUPS egg whites (from 18 eggs) or 16 oz prepared liquid egg whites

- 3 TABLESPOONS nutritional yeast

- 1 ½ TEASPOONS Better than Bouillon No-Chicken Base

- 1 ½ TEASPOONS sweet rice flour or cornstarch

- ½ TEASPOON onion powder

- Nonstick spray (optional)

- ½ TEASPOON paprika for garnish

- ½ CUP cherry tomatoes halved for garnish

Instructions

- Preheat oven to 350ºF.

- In a large, heavy-bottomed saute pan over medium heat, combine mushrooms, zucchini, yellow onion, dried tomatoes, 2 teaspoons of the thyme, garlic, salt, and 1/4 teaspoon of the pepper with ½ cup water.

- Cook, stirring frequently, until vegetables are soft and onions are translucent, 8–10 minutes.

- Add kale. Cook, stirring frequently, until kale is tender, about 5 minutes. Add up to 2 more tablespoons water if necessary, if vegetables seem dry or are starting to brown. Any extra water should evaporate by the time the kale is tender.

- In a blender, combine egg whites, nutritional yeast, bouillon base, sweet rice flour or cornstarch, onion powder, remaining teaspoon of thyme and ¼ teaspoon of pepper.

• Blend at medium speed for 10 seconds, until ingredients are well mixed.

• Lightly spray an 8 x 8-in glass baking pan with nonstick spray, or use a nonstick baking pan.

• Spread vegetables evenly over bottom of baking pan. Pour egg mixture evenly over vegetables.

• Sprinkle lightly with paprika.

• Cover pan with aluminum foil.

• Bake frittata for 20 minutes. Remove foil and continue to bake until frittata is set in the middle and edges are lightly browned, about 10 to 15 minutes. Remove frittata from the oven.

- Let sit for at least 10 minutes before serving.

- Cut frittata into four 4 x 4-in squares. Garnish each square with tomato halves.

Ornish Tofu Teryaki

Preparation time

50 minutes

INGREDIENTS

- 1 CUP unseasoned sake

- 1 CUP mirin (sweet rice wine)

- ¾ CUP water

- 1/3 CUP reduced-sodium tamari or soy sauce

- 1 TABLESPOON fresh ginger root peeled and finely chopped

- 1 TABLESPOON fresh garlic pressed or minced

- 1 ½ LB extra-firm tofu cut into ½ inch cubes (6 cups)

- 4 CUPS fresh shiitake, cremini, or white mushrooms, or a combination stems removed, quartered (1 lb)

- 1 CUP onion peeled and coarsely chopped

- 3 TABLESPOONS sweet rice flour or cornstarch

- ¼ CUP water

- 1 LARGE HEAD broccoli or 4 cups florets

- 1/3 CUP scallions thinly sliced (optional)

- 3 CUPS cooked brown rice (optional, for serving)

Instructions

- Preheat oven to 350°F. In a large bowl, combine sake, mirin, 3/4 cup water, tamari or soy sauce, ginger and garlic. Add the tofu, stirring to coat. Marinate for at least 30 minutes. (Tofu can be marinated for several hours, or overnight.) After marinating, strain the tofu, reserving the marinade.

- Line a baking sheet with parchment paper. Spread tofu cubes evenly over baking sheet. Bake until tofu is lightly browned, about 30 minutes. Remove from oven and set aside.

• Place a steamer basket in a saucepan and add water to just below the bottom of steamer basket. Over high heat, bring water to a boil. Add broccoli florets. Cover and cook until broccoli is just tender, about 3 minutes. Remove basket and rinse broccoli quickly with cold water. Drain and set aside.

• In a large, heavy-bottomed saute pan over medium-high heat, bring mushrooms, onions and 3/4 cup of the reserved tofu marinade to a simmer. Simmer, stirring frequently, until mushrooms are softened and onions are translucent, about 7–10 minutes.

• Add remaining marinade, bring to a simmer and cook for 3 to 4 minutes to evaporate the alcohol from the mixture.

- In a small bowl, whisk sweet rice flour or cornstarch with ¼ cup water until smooth. Whisk this mixture into the mushrooms and cook until glossy and thickened, 1–2 minutes. Add tofu, broccoli, and scallions, if using, reserving about 1 tablespoon of scallions for garnish. Cook, stirring frequently until tofu and vegetables are heated through.

- Serve over rice, if using. Garnish with reserved scallions.

Lentil Soup

Preparation time

1 hour

Ingredients

- 1 pound lentils

- 1 bay leaf

- 3 large carrots, peeled and sliced

- 2 stalks celery, chopped

- 1 large onion, chopped

- 1/2 teaspoon cumin powder

- 2 cups crushed tomatoes (fresh or canned)

- 2 tablespoons extra-virgin olive oil

- Salt and pepper to taste

- Vinegar (red wine, cider or balsamic, optional)

Instructions

1. Pick over lentils to remove any stones, dirt, or other foreign objects.

2. Rinse them well in cold water and place in a large pot with enough cold water to cover lentils by 6 inches. Add the bay leaf.

3. Bring to a boil, skim off foam, lower heat, and boil gently, partially covered, until lentils are just tooth-tender, 20-30 minutes.

4. Add carrots, celery, cumin and onion to the lentils. Cook partially covered till carrots are tender, about 20-30 minutes.

5. Add crushed tomatoes, olive oil, and salt and pepper to taste. Simmer, partially covered, until lentils become very creamy and soft. Stir occasionally and add boiling water if necessary to prevent sticking.

6. Remove bay leaf before serving. If you like, stir in a little vinegar just before serving.

Ornish Carrot Cupcakes with Non-fat Maple frosting

Preparation time

1 hour 5 minutes

INGREDIENTS

For Cupcakes:

• Nonstick cooking spray

• 2 ¼ CUPS whole-wheat pastry flour

• 1/3 CUP brown sugar

- 2 TEASPOONS baking powder

- 1 TEASPOON powdered stevia

- 1 ½ TEASPOONS cinnamon

- ¾ TEASPOON fine sea salt

- ¼ TEASPOON nutmeg

- 1/8 TEASPOON ground cloves

- 1 TABLESPOON ground flax meal

- 1 TABLESPOON water

- 1 ½ CUPS carrot grated, 3 medium carrots

- ¾ CUP unsweetened almond milk

- ½ CUP unsweetened applesauce

- 2 TEASPOONS vanilla extract

For Frosting:

1. ONE 8-OZ PACKAGE nonfat cream cheese at room temperature

2. 1/3 CUP pure maple syrup

3. 1 TEASPOON vanilla extract

Instructions

- Preheat oven to 375ºF. Lightly spray a muffin pan with nonstick cooking spray, or line cups with paper liners and lightly spray liners.

- In a large bowl, mix together whole wheat pastry flour, brown sugar, baking powder, stevia, cinnamon, salt, nutmeg, and cloves.

- In a medium bowl, mix flax meal with water. Let sit until water is absorbed, 1 to 2 minutes.

Add carrots, almond milk, applesauce, and vanilla extract.

- Stir the carrot mixture into the flour mixture. Mix well.

- Spoon 1/4 cup batter into each muffin cup.

- Bake for 30 to 35 minutes, until a toothpick inserted in the center comes out clean.

- Remove from oven and let cool on a rack.

- Place muffin pan on a rack and let cupcakes cool in the pan for 10 minutes, until cupcakes pull away slightly from the edges of the muffin cups.

- Remove cupcakes from pan and let cool completely on a rack. Cupcakes should be completely cool before frosting.

• To make the frosting, in a small bowl, combine cream cheese, maple syrup, and vanilla extract.

• Using a hand-held electric mixer, beat on high speed until smooth.

• To frost cupcakes, spread a heaping tablespoon of frosting evenly across the top of each cupcake just before serving. These are best enjoyed the day they are made.

Ornish Mac 'n Cheez

Preparation time

25 minutes

INGREDIENTS

For Sauce:

1. 1 TABLESPOON arrowroot or cornstarch

2. 1 TABLESPOON water

3. 2 CUPS unsweetened soy milk

4. ¼ CUP nutritional yeast plus more for garnish

5. ¼ CUP white miso paste or white chickpea miso

6. 2 TABLESPOONS tomato paste

7. 2 TEASPOONS onion powder

8. 1 TEASPOON dry mustard

For Pasta:

• ONE 8.8-OZ PACKAGE whole grain or gluten-free penne pasta, or preferred shape

• 4 CUPS broccoli florets (8 oz)

- 1/8 TEASPOON freshly ground pepper

- Paprika or smoked paprika for garnish

Instructions

- Bring a large, heavy-bottomed pot of water to a boil.

- In a small bowl, whisk arrowroot or cornstarch with 1 tablespoon water until dissolved.

- In a small saucepan over medium heat, whisk together soy milk, nutritional yeast, white miso, tomato paste, onion powder, and dry mustard. Bring to a simmer.

- Reduce heat to medium-low and whisk in arrowroot or cornstarch mixture. Cook, whisking frequently, until sauce thickens, 2–3 minutes. Cover and set aside to keep warm.

• Cook pasta in pot of boiling water according to package instructions. Cook until pasta is cooked through but still firm to the bite ("al dente").

• While pasta is cooking, place a vegetable steamer basket in a saucepan and add water to just below bottom of steamer basket. Over medium heat, bring water to a boil. Add broccoli. Cover and steam until broccoli is just tender but still bright green, 4 to 5 minutes.

• Drain pasta and broccoli and return to the empty pasta pot. Add the warm sauce and toss to coat. Garnish with a sprinkle of paprika. Serve with additional nutritional yeast.

Un-Do It Tacos

Preparation time

30 minutes

INGREDIENTS

1. 6 corn tortillas

2. 1 cup onion diced to ¼ inch

3. 1 cup yellow corn fresh or frozen

4. 1 cup water

5. 1 envelope spicy taco seasoning mix, suggested brand: "Simply Organic" Southwest Taco

6. 12 ounce package ground veggie crumbles, suggested brand: "Yves" MEXICAN SLAW (optional)

7. 3 cups green cabbage finely sliced

8. 3 cups purple cabbage finely sliced

9. 12 ounce package silken tofu

10. ¾ cup picante sauce mild, suggested brand: Pace

11. 1/4 teaspoon salt (optional)

12. Garnish (optional):

13. Fat free cheddar cheese grated, suggested brand: LifeTime

14. Chopped cilantro

INSTRUCTIONS

• Simmer the onion, corn, water and seasoning mix together, in a pan over medium heat, until the onions are translucent.

• Add and mix in the Veggie

• Ground and cook the taco filling for a few minutes, stirring frequently for no more than 5 minutes.

• While the taco filling is cooking, prepare the Mexican slaw.

• Blend the tofu and the picante sauce in a blender or food processor and mix this dressing with the thinly sliced cabbage.

- Heat the tortillas and serve them with the taco filling, the Mexican slaw, (optional) nonfat cheddar cheese and cilantro.

Ornish Lentil Loaf

Preparation time

2 hours

INGREDIENTS

1. 1 CUP uncooked short grain brown rice

2. 1 CUP uncooked French black or green lentils

3. 8 OZ frozen spinach thawed

4. 1 ½ CUPS onion diced

5. 1 ½ CUPS carrots grated

6. 1 TABLESPOON garlic pressed or minced

7. 2 TABLESPOONS Bragg Liquid Aminos, divided

8. 1 TABLESPOON fresh thyme, divided or 1 ½ teaspoons dried thyme, divided

9. 1 TEASPOON dried oregano

10. 1/2 TEASPOON freshly ground pepper, divided

11. 1 CUP water, divided plus more as needed

12. Smoky Chipotle Ketchup (see description, above, for recipe link)

Instructions

• Preheat oven to 375ºF. Prepare rice and lentils according to package instructions. (The rice and lentils can be prepared up to two days ahead of time, and refrigerated until needed.)

• Place thawed spinach in a colander in the sink or over a deep bowl. Using your hands, squeeze or press spinach vigorously to remove excess liquid. Continue to squeeze and press spinach until it is almost dry; excess liquid left in the spinach will make a soggy loaf. Once drained, you should have about ¾ cup of spinach. Set aside.

• In a large saute pan over medium-low heat, sauté the onions, carrots, garlic, 1 tablespoon of the Bragg liquid aminos, 1 1/2 teaspoons of the fresh thyme, oregano, ¼ teaspoon of the pepper, and ½ cup of the water. Stirring frequently, saute until onions are translucent, 7–10 minutes.

• In a large bowl, combine the cooked rice and the lentils with the onion mixture. Add the remaining 1 tablespoon liquid aminos, 1 1/2 teaspoons fresh thyme and 1/4 teaspoon pepper. Mix well.

• Spoon half of the rice mixture (about 3 1/2 cups) into a food processor. Pulse, adding ½ cup water as needed, until mixture is a thick paste. Mix this back into the remaining lentil mixture. Add the spinach and stir well to combine.

• Line a baking sheet with parchment paper. Form and tightly pack lentil mixture into a loaf 2 inches high and 9 inches long. Bake for about 40 minutes, or until it is lightly browned and crisped on the top. Remove from oven and spread ½ cup Smoky Chipotle Ketchup evenly on top. Let cook for an additional 10 minutes. Remove from oven. (If you have an instant-read or digital thermometer, the internal temperature should read 165–170ºF.)

- Let loaf rest for 10 minutes before slicing and serving.

Pumpkin Pie

Preparation time

35 minutes

Ingredients

FOR CRUST:

- 9 OZ (ABOUT 14) lowfat graham crackers approved Reversal brand, such as Nabisco low fat

- ⅓ CUP PLUS 1 TABLESPOON unsweetened soy, oat or flax milk

FOR FILLING:

1. 1/2 CUP (ABOUT 6 DATES, OR 3 OZ) pitted medjool dates

2. 1 1/2 CUPS unsweetened soy, oat, or flax milk

3. 2 TABLESPOONS agar agar (sea vegetable flakes)

4. ONE 15-OZ CAN unsweetened pumpkin puree

5. 3 TABLESPOONS flax meal

6. 1 1/2 TEASPOONS cinnamon

7. 1 TEASPOON vanilla extract

8. 1 TEASPOON ground ginger

9. 1/8 TEASPOON ground cloves

10. 1/2 TEASPOON fine sea salt

Instructions

• Preheat oven to 325ºF. To make the crust, crumble graham crackers into the bowl of a food processor fitted with the metal blade. Pulse until crackers form fine crumbs. Add soy milk and pulse until mixture holds its form when pressed.

- Using your fingers, press the mixture evenly over the bottom and sides of a 9-inch pie pan. Place the pan in the oven and bake until crust is lightly browned, about 10 to 12 minutes. Remove from oven and set on a rack to cool.

- To make the filling, place dates in a small bowl with 1/2 cup hot water. Cover bowl and let sit until dates are softened, about 10 minutes. Strain, reserving 1/4 cup of the date-soaking liquid.

- In a medium-sized, heavy-bottomed saucepan over medium heat, combine nondairy milk and agar agar. Bring to a simmer, whisking frequently. Reduce heat and cook, whisking frequently, until agar agar is completely dissolved, about 5 minutes.

- Remove from heat. Whisk in softened dates, reserved 1/4 cup of date-soaking liquid, pumpkin, flax meal, cinnamon, vanilla, ginger, cloves, and salt. Working in batches if necessary, pour pumpkin mixture into a blender, being careful to fill blender no more than two-thirds full. On low speed, blend mixture until smooth.

- Pour filling into prepared crust. (You may not need all the filling. Pour any extra into a ramekin or serving dish. Chill and serve as pumpkin custard.) Place pie in refrigerator and chill for several hours before serving. Pie will firm up and set as it cools. If you like your pumpkin pie served warm, cover the chilled pie with aluminum foil and warm in a 300°F oven for 10 minutes.

Ornish Edamole

Preparation time

10 minutes

INGREDIENTS

1. 2 CUPS frozen shelled edamame thawed

2. ¾ CUP silken tofu

3. 1–2 CLOVES garlic pressed or minced to taste

4. ½ TEASPOON ground cumin

5. 2 TABLESPOONS fresh lime juice

6. ½ –1 TEASPOON fine sea salt to taste

7. ¼ TEASPOON lime zest (optional)

8. 1 small tomato seeded and diced (optional)

9. ¼ CUP cilantro chopped (optional)

10. 2 TABLESPOONS red onion diced (optional)

11. 2-3 DASHES hot sauce, green or red (optional)

Instructions

1. In a food processor, combine edamame, tofu, garlic, cumin, lime juice, and 1/2 teaspoon of the salt.

2. Pulse until ingredients are blended to desired texture; you can stop while mixture is still chunky and coarse or continue to process into a smooth, thick paste.

3. Use a rubber spatula to scrape down the sides as needed.

4. Transfer mixture to a bowl. Taste for seasoning and add additional salt as needed. Stir in lime zest, diced tomato, cilantro, red onion, and/or hot sauce, if using.

5. Serve as a dip with an assortment of raw vegetables and fat-free whole grain crackers, or use as a sandwich spread.

Ornish Spinach and Mushroom Egg White Scramble Recipe

Preparation time

20 minutes

INGREDIENTS

1. 1 ½ CUPS onions diced

2. 4 CUPS white mushrooms sliced

3. ¼ CUP water

4. ½ TEASPOON turmeric

5. ½ TEASPOON garlic powder

6. ¼ TEASPOON freshly ground pepper, divided

7. 1/8 TEASPOON fine sea salt

8. 1 ½ CUPS egg whites from approximately 8 eggs

9. 4 CUPS baby spinach leaves

10. Smoked paprika for garnish (optional)

Instructions

- In a large 12-inch sauté pan over medium heat, combine onions, mushrooms, water, turmeric, garlic powder, 1/8 teaspoon of the pepper, and salt.

- Cook, stirring occasionally, until mushrooms are tender, onions are translucent, and all moisture has evaporated, about 7 to 10 minutes.

- Add egg whites and remaining 1/8 teaspoon pepper.

- Cook, stirring frequently, until egg whites are opaque.

- Just before the egg whites are fully cooked, fold in the spinach. Continue cooking until spinach is wilted and any excess liquid has evaporated. Taste for seasoning, adding additional salt if desired.

- Sprinkle with smoked paprika, if using. Serve immediately.

Made in the USA
Coppell, TX
10 April 2022

76341643R10075